T0367969

Why You DON'T Want to be a Doctor

Why You DON'T Want to be a Doctor

Real Stories from an Insider

Dr. Y

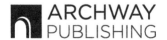

ARCHWAY
PUBLISHING

Archway Publishing books may be ordered
through booksellers or by contacting:

Archway Publishing
1663 Liberty Drive
Bloomington, IN 47403
www.archwaypublishing.com
844-669-3957

ISBN: 978-1-6657-6505-3 (sc)
ISBN: 978-1-6657-6506-0 (e)

Library of Congress Control Number: 2024917257

Print information available on the last page.

Archway Publishing rev. date: 04/07/2025

Contents

Prelude

While writing this book I have looked back on my career as a Board-Certified Internal Medicine/ Hospitalist Medicine Physician. I have noted my perspective has changed greatly. I no longer laugh at the jokes I previously found funny. And, although I promised myself I would never allow medicine to change me, it has.

I hope you enjoy sharing with me, these moments of laughter, toil, and tears.

The Journey Comes With a Price

After all the years of undergraduate B.S. I had finished my sociology classes, I had completed my interpersonal communications classes, I had taken numerous required gym classes, and at long last I was done with that crazy interpretive dance class! I had graduated with my degree in B.S., I was well rounded, and I had a pretty little price tag to show for it.

I had studied long and hard for my MCAT, which I passed after paying thousands of dollars to MCAT prep classes and for MCAT prep books. I then paid even more thousands of dollars to apply to medical schools across the country. When I received my letters for interviews, I gladly laid down my credit card, for a continued financial outgo, to catch the next flight out! Hotels, food, and flights, were just additive to my undergraduate education costs, my testing fees, my application processing fees, my information service carrier fees, my transcript fees, and every other charge the medical school application process could throw my way. Everyone wanted a piece of the financial pie, and boy did they get it!

To this day I remember receiving the letter confirming my acceptance. I was so overjoyed that I had been brought into the fold, I had been accepted into "the club".

"Dear Ms. Y,

We are happy to inform you that you have been accepted into our prestigious medical program. Kindly send your deposit for $3000.00 to hold your accepted spot. We regret to inform you, that if we do not receive your payment within 10 days, we will be unable to hold your spot any longer and we will be forced to accept a less qualified student in your place. Again, congratulations, and we are looking forward to seeing you in May."

My answer of course was, do you accept visa?

The Cadaver

Prior to the first day of medical school, I arranged to meet with some of the other students that were going to be in my class. We were all so excited to be there, anticipating our future studies, listening to stories from previous medical students, bonding with those who were about to share in our misery, and obtaining critical pearls as we were able.

We soon discovered from this opportunity that a very important key to our learning possibilities would rely on the quality of our very near future, A&P cadaver. Cadavers with too little fat, or that were to old, would dry out and would not last throughout the semester. Thus leaving you with no real tissue example for dissection. Cadavers with too much fat would make dissection a nightmare, as a one hour dissection could easily turn into a four hour saga, should too much adipose tissue remain in your path. Thus, the integrity of this cadaver could be the catapult that would ensure our A&P success!

Our answer to the pressing conundrum was clearly that we would need to take action and formulate a detailed plan immediately! We all returned home that evening with homework. One of us was to find the hours we would be able to access the A&P Lab without inquiring minds. Another of us would research when the cadavers would be delivered to the lab and when the first A&P Lab was scheduled. The third member would attempt to determine how the cadavers were to be assigned to us.

The following day we met again, this time with the vital pieces to mold our plan. We had found that on the first day of classes we would all be allowed to pick our cadavers, but that the cadavers would be covered in bags, obscuring the quality, age, sex, or size of each cadaver. Second, the cadavers were being delivered to the lab this very day, with the first day of classes following in the morning. Finally, and most importantly, the professors and lab assistants would be attending a dinner at 7:00-8:00pm vacating the lab for this period and allowing us a small window to choose an excellent specimen. We agreed to meet at 6:00pm and arrive together at the school, then wait around the corner from the lab until the momentous opportunity arrived.

By 7:15pm our lab had become eerily silent. We ventured from our deftly chosen hiding places and made quick work of our task at hand. In the far back of the room we found an amazing discovery. This cadaver was a mid-weight, athletic, middle aged man that was, for lack of a better word, perfect! We noted his location carefully. In a room of 70 cadavers, we did not wish to take a risk in misplacing him!

Upon returning to the lab the next morning, we waited with bated breath. We thought to ourselves how our fellow classmates had no idea what was about to befall them and how brilliant we had been to complete our mission the night prior. We anxiously fidgeted back and forth, we bit our nails, we twisted our hair, until we heard the command "Please walk to a cadaver and stand next to it". All three of us literally ran to our cadaver on the other end of the room. As we ran, our other classmates followed suit, running to the nearest cadaver they could find.

Unbelievably, the three of us made it to our cadaver and rejoiced. It must have been odd to our fellow classmates to watch us all celebrating such an event.

After everyone else had found a cadaver, the lab assistant ordered us to remove our cadaver's body bag and to examine our year's learning subject. As we began to unzip our bag, we noticed something wasn't quite right. Our cadaver had bloated overnight, or maybe we didn't remember him being just a little larger? It was a complete shock to find that our cadaver was a 450lb woman in her 70s! As a matter of fact, she was the heaviest cadaver in the room! After the Professors had finished their dinner the night prior, they had returned to the lab and moved all of the cadavers to different positions based on gender and age.

Every A&P Lab day following resulted in the three of us literally soaked in fat, status post dissection. Greasy and smelly we would have to head to the showers, of course this would be after everyone else had left the lab, with our dissections taking so much longer. If we had been caught picking out our cadaver that fateful night, there could not have been a worse punishment than the one we had inflicted on ourselves!

Hooked on Phonics
Worked for Me

One of the most difficult challenges of medical school is the sheer quantity of memorization. The amount of information you must learn in such a short amount of time requires you to use your time wisely. The key is to understanding what study method works for you and finding that out quickly is paramount to your very survival. Auditory learners, visual learners, and practical skills learners all must employ different learning techniques. Some people use flash cards, which I did, but only for quick review. Some people form note pools, which I attempted, but the time required printing pretty notes for other people seemed to work against me. Others NEVER missed a lecture. This was a thing I knew better than to do from my undergraduate studies, as I am not an auditory learner. Some tape each lecture and listen to it later. A technique I found to require too much time. Some work in groups only, usually practical skills learners do best this way. This is just social time for me, I can't retain this way. Finally, some have to read the content for themselves. These are visual learners. This is the most boring and lonely way to learn, which of course is my required study and retaining method.

Also of importance you must learn that study time is exactly that. Study time is sacred! You are embarking on an all exclusive vacation to the library/ your study room/ your quiet place. No unexpected family visitors or spur of the moment flighty ideas from your friends or colleagues should tear you away. It is difficult. It is exhausting. There is a reason about half of my original medical school class did not graduate with me. You must remain totally committed to study.

There are of course additional pearls for memorization. As I have always said, hooked on phonics worked for me. My colleagues and I devised catchy phrases and songs to commit large amounts of otherwise unrelated information to memory. The cranial nerves had an interesting pneumonic, that I will spare you, but that you will positively learn if you attend medical school. One of my favorite songs was memorizing the Lady Gaga twist "gitchy gitchy fascia lata". I also enjoyed the Harry Potter spell for "Corona Radiata".

Truly, the more you are able to incorporate these odd terms into your familiar daily life, the easier it is to remember them when you are exhausted and you have had 20 cups of coffee.

Back Up

If you have ever visited a career counselor you will know that it is paramount to have a plan B. Yes of course, we all dream of plan A. We all strive for plan A. We type A personalities like only to consider plan A. However, in the world in which we live, a plan B and maybe even a plan C are prudent necessities.

When I was accepted into medical school, I was fortunate to have the ability to choose a school. I fell in love with the school, the people, and the opportunities of the area. However, I had no idea what I was truly in store for.

Medical school was hard. It required constant studying and testing, testing and studying, did I mention the studying and testing? Whereas in college I had been heads above the other students, in medical school, I was just one of the run of the mill students.

I hadn't gotten dumber, but I sure felt like I had. Mastering the amount of information required to learn in a condensed time period was impossible at best.

During many of my study sessions, I would study in my car. My car provided privacy, removal from social interaction, but most importantly isolation. Which was required for my material retention and regurgitation.

I would commonly drive my car to an isolated spot next to a bird sanctuary. Sitting next to this bird sanctuary was a National Forrest Building. I remember telling myself on multiple accounts....... "If I fail this upcoming test, I can always be a Forrest Ranger", my loosely formulated plan B. I never had enough spare time to make a plan C.

When I graduated medical school, I remember looking toward the National Forrest Building and thinking, thank goodness, what does a Forest Ranger do anyway?

Vegas: Sex, Drugs and Gambling

If you have never visited Las Vegas, I would say you are missing something. However, the truth of the matter is that the only things you would be missing would be legal prostitution, gambling, substance abuse, high speed racing on the freeway, the second poorest water quality in the nation, and drunken brawling. For a bachelor party, it has all the amenities. For a drive thru wedding, Vegas can hook you up. But for a residency program, it rocks!

As a resident, you are able to see so much. You have patients from all over the globe, with a multitude of different histories of medical care. You have the visitors that come for the gluttony, who overindulge in the seven deadly sins. You have an enormous homeless population with no or very poor previous medical care. And of course you have the MMA guys who come in after doing the craziest crap to each other. Vegas is a great place to learn medicine.

Of course this opportunity is not such for all residents. Some residents have a propensity to distraction, which can become problematic in Vegas. I did have fellow residents who failed out secondary to substance abuse. Other fellow residents gambled away their futures. Sadly, I even had a fellow resident who died from too much of "all that Vegas has to offer".

That being said, when you choose your residency program, it is important not only to consider the program with the big name, or the one your family went to. You must factor yourself into the equation of where YOU will best excel.

Many residency programs will meet your check boxes on paper, but when you arrive to evaluate them, they fall short substantially. My recommendation would be, when you are in medical school and you have the opportunity to evaluate programs across the country for your future residency position, do not take this lightly. Arrange rotations across the country that will allow you the closest experience to actual residency there, before becoming a resident. You want to arrange "audition rotations" in all of the programs that pique your interest. This is usually in your third and fourth year of medical school. These audition rotations inform the program that you are interested in attending their program as a resident and they will put you to work. Plan for 120 hour weeks, this is not a joke.

Work hard. Show up early. Stay late. Don't ever complain. Yada… yada… yada. But remember to look at the programs closely yourself. You are "interviewing" while you are rotating, but the programs are also applying for a job with you. This is for your education, your base as a physician.

Although medical school is important for integrating your didactics, internship and residency are the brick and mortar upon which your entire practice will rest as an attending. This relatively small amount of time, roughly 4 to 5 years, for you to practice as a physician, in such an information rich environment, will not be an opportunity that will arise again. If you shortcut these years, you will never be able to go back to replace what you missed and eventually when you become an attending, it will be readily apparent by your patients and your peers, that you do not have a solid foundation. This is the time to get it right!

When on your audition rotations you must talk to the residents already in the program and ask them their opinion of their internship/residency program. If the residents there already have some real concerns, pay attention.

Pick the things that are important to you inside the program and outside of the program too. Will you be happy living where it rains every day if you get seasonal affective disorder? Will you be able to focus on your studies in a place where you are going to be required to have 4 roommates to pay the rent? If you have a family, will they have their needs met at the location of your choice? There is no one size fits all residency program. Be certain to consider your own limitations/strengths for your personal success.

The Dreaded Dr. S

The Dreaded Dr. S was a legend in my residency program. The nurses, the other residents, and even the attendings warned me of him from the start. He had ties with the mafia. His friends were the judges in town. He knew everyone and everything and you did not want to mess with him, much less get on his s**t list.

He was a very intelligent attending who did nothing but probe in depth concerning every internal medicine topic, I had never heard of. When I rounded with him I physically carried a stack of books. I had books in all of my pockets of my white coat. I had a clip board where I fit more books inside. I had a stack of books on top of the clip board I carried in my arms. I was a walking library!

The Dreaded Dr. S would pimp as he probed and

he would question without missing a step. He would walk toward a patient's room, while asking a question prior to entering, he would examine the patient and speak with them, and then he would pick up from the same sentence, many times mid sentence, upon exiting the room.

The "Dreaded Dr. S" would ask, "Dr. Y, why do we breathe"? Being eager, at the beginning I would say the first thing that came to my mind. ... Which was always wrong by the way, and for which I would receive an over the glasses stare from the Dreaded Dr. S to let me know that I was not only ignorant, but that I was clearly also stupid and incompetent. Even after all of the hours spent diligently cramming my didactics, I was pond scum. Soon I realized that if I held my tongue, looked through my books, and thought out each question slowly prior to answering, I would not only answer correctly, but I would learn why it was so.

The Dreaded Dr.S did have a method to his treachery, which eventually served me well. However, there are times to this day that I look over my shoulder to be certain The Dreaded Dr. S is not looking over his readers at me.

Patients Lie

A disturbing reality of helping people is it can be difficult to get the truth. No patient wants to look their doctor in the eye and say, "I put that up my butt because it felt good." The usual response is "I don't know how that got there."

Because of this paradigm you must always remember, patients lie.

One night in the ER I had been called to admit a patient with suicidal ideation. This patient had been brought in to the hospital by the police after his girlfriend had the police beat down his front door. The police had been told this gentleman was suicidal and he would not come to the door. Thus, being the heroes they truly are, they bashed down the door and justly drug the man from his bedroom.

After talking with this suicidal gentleman, he explained to me that he had been fighting with his girlfriend and that he was not trying to kill himself, nor was he suicidal. He swore to me that his intentions were not to harm himself, but actually to get high. This gentleman had a history of heroin abuse and he had just been released from rehab. He stated that he "fell off the wagon" and he had injected himself with heroin on this evening. The police corroborated this story stating they did find him with a needle in his arm.

The gentleman asked if he could please return home, stating again that he was not suicidal, and that he wished to follow up with his own psychiatrist in the morning for continued assistance with his drug addiction. The police were planning on giving this gentleman a break and were not arresting him for drug charges. As the gentleman's story appeared credible and his mother came to the ER to pick him up after she was allowed full disclosure to the nights activities, I released this gentleman to his mother's care.

One week later, this same gentleman returned to the ER with two broken ankles, and oh by the way, a rope ligature around his neck.

Always remember, patients lie.

My First Code

When you become a medical student, one of the first experiences you look forward to greatly is participating in your first code. It is an event that you do not know how you will react to and although you look forward with anticipation, you additionally experience a bit of dread. You wonder if you will not know what to do. Maybe you will freeze. Perhaps you will kill someone. All sobering, tortuous thoughts, and you do not know how you will react until you actually are there.

My first code occurred when I was a 3rd year medical student. I was rounding with my attending, the "Dreaded Dr. S.", when he stopped walking, looked directly at a patient in the ICU, and asked me, "What's wrong with that patient"? Knowing nothing of the patient's history, I quickly peered at him from the doorway. He appeared to be resting and I said nothing, as I had no clue as to any problem readily apparent.

The "Dreaded Dr. S" quickly shoved me aside as he told me, "this patient is not breathing! " Dr. S. pulled the code alarm on the wall and before I could even blink, 5 ICU techs came running into the room. As a finely tuned machine, they brought clipboards, and medications, and crash carts, oh my!

Compressions were started and blood began to spurt everywhere. The "Dreaded Dr. S" paged the surgeon who had just completed cardiovascular surgery on this patient 2 days prior. But as luck would have it, he happened to be right down the hall when the code alarm sounded. He also ran to the patient's bedside and he was pissed when he got there.

It was a complete fiasco from that point forward. The finely tuned machine began to fall apart as the surgeon yelled, "Get the F'ing blood. The O negative F'ing blood. Where the F is the rapid transfuser? Why does the patient not have the F'ing defibrillation pads on yet? "

Techs turned on one another. One tech attempted

to put defibrillation pads on the patient and another screamed for her to get out of the way while she was continuing compressions. One tech headed to the patients head and grabbed an ambu bag that had not yet been hooked into the wall for oxygen. One tech ran from the room frantic. The remaining tech and I both stood with our eyes wide and our jaws dropped, not able to believe what we were seeing.

The surgeon continued to yell orders throughout the entire code which only caused further mayhem. "F'ing this and F'ing that". Blood F'ing flew here and blood F'ing flew there. The whole room looked like a crime scene.

Needless to say, after 60 minutes of discombobulation, the time of death was called. At that point everyone in the room had been spattered with blood. The surgeon threw down his blood soaked scrub top onto the floor and headed down the hall where I could still hear him yelling "F'ing this and F'ing that".

That day has lingered in my memory for quite some time, and although the patient died in that code, I did learn something positive from that experience.

To this day I have never yelled in a code, much less yelled the F word. I learned that keeping a calm head and communicating effectively with my staff allowed for the well oiled machine to function. I found if I respected my staff, and I gave them the opportunity to excel, they would do just that, working as a team. Because after all, isn't saving lives what it is F'ing all about anyway?

A Good ID Doc is Worth His Weight in Platinum

On my second night as an intern I can remember one of the scariest events in my entire training. I had a very pleasant 18 year old girl come in covered from head to toe with an erythematous, lacy rash. She had a fever of 102.0 and was beginning to slur her words. The interns had all been informed of an undiagnosed viral condition that was affecting the younger patients with this similar symptomology and that a 16 year old boy had died of this condition two weeks prior.

My girl had been at a slumber party with all of her friends the night before, she had eaten different foods than usual, and her family had just returned from a trip outside of the country. All of these risk factors I took into consideration as my girl progressively worsened. I had examined her, I had placed her on broad spectrum antibiotics, I was aggressively hydrating her, I had imaged her, I had reviewed all of her medications that could be complicating her picture, I had ordered a tox screen, a hematology panel, a rheumatology panel, conducted an LP, and cultures of body. I had considered and worked up multiple zebras, as all her laboratory values remained normal, she continued to decline. Her temperature progressed to 104.0, she became tachycardic, hypotensive, and incoherent.

It was at that point that I knew if this girl had a chance of living I had to go to a higher power! My chief resident was swamped with other critical cases, so I informed him that I needed to call ID. He nodded at me half way as he rushed to another room. I then headed to the consultant list and dialed the Attending Infectious Disease Physician.

"Dr. M, Hello sir. My name is Dr. Y. I am the intern on call this evening. I have a very sick patient I need your help with. I am sorry to wake you at 2am. Could you please assist me with this case?"

Dr. M replied, in a perturbed and obviously

somulent tone "Dr. Y, I am not on call this evening. How did you get my number?"

My mind raced as I apologized profusely awaiting my intense persecution. "Doctor Y, you will now be on call Q2, you will happily admit every psych admit that comes through our doors, you will perform all cavity searches of our altered patients, you will present a case at morning report daily, and you will never ever make the mistake of calling me again, especially at 2am!"

To my complete amazement Dr. M actually replied, "Tell me about the patient."

After swallowing my tongue, I ran down the complete list of my girl's condition. I included her history, her precise progression, and I quickly pointed out the conditions I had been able to rule out. Dr. M agreed with my textbook assessment/treatment, but he did inform me that there were Eight other medications/treatments that he wanted me to add emergently or that my girl would most certainly die.

I quickly placed a central line and ran to the lab to facilitate the processing of the many abnormal orders. I had everything hanging within 20 minutes.

Another 20 minutes later she turned the corner. Her heart rate slowed, she became normotensive, her fever curve decreased, and within an hour she was talking again!

By 3:00am Dr M was at my girl's bedside, verifying that his orders had been carried out to the number. He meticulously examined the patient, reviewed the chart, and then he headed over to me. "Dr. Y, This is the virus that killed our 16 year old two weeks ago. Even though you were following the textbook treatment to the letter, this girl would have died if you hadn't given me a call. Nice work!"

To this day I still have the actual list that gracious Dr. M ordered me to give. You never know when you might need to save a teenager. Of course Dr. M is still on my speed dial!

Don't Forget to Pay the Prostitute

Many times when you are working as a discrete, HIPPA bound, trustworthy physician, you will be amazed at the facts patients will be unwilling to tell you until they have no way of denying it. Multiple "accidental" excuses are found for foreign bodies which are incidentally found only through imaging or physical examination.

One such instance readily comes to my mind when I think back about working in Nevada. A patient presented to me in the ER complaining of BL knee pain. He stated the pain had started about 2 days prior and that he awoke with the pain, which was searing. He stated the pain had been worsening since that time, to the point where he could no longer walk.

After a thorough examination I found the patient's anterior and posterior drawer signs to be negative. No ligamentous abnormality was apparent. Neither knees demonstrated erythema nor calor. However, the patient cried out in pain when I examined his genitals. His external meatus was fire-engine red and there was something visually noted within his urethra.

10 minutes later I had obtained a cystoscope which elucidated a very feathery, green abnormality. With a very long set of forceps a green onion was withdrawn from this man's penis, with the bulb of the onion last.

Only at that point did the patient admit to me that he had visited a prostitute two days earlier. He had been intimate with this same prostitute three months prior to this latest visit and at that time he had skipped out on paying her. He thought the prostitute would forget his prior transgression, but apparently she had not. When he returned two days ago she was very friendly, she gave him free alcoholic beverages, and from his fuzzy memory, she and her friend had brought in the onions for "sexual stimulation."

My advice to him at that juncture was, Bactrim DS PO BID and next time, don't forget to pay the prostitute.

The Gamma

Every residency program has at least one good practical joker. The guy that farts and burps just aren't funny enough to. The guy that is always planning his next prank. He is likable to most everyone. He has a quit wit. He is believable when he lies. He makes an impressive doctor!

In my residency program Dr. A. was our prankster extraordinaire. He had one prank that stills brings tears to my eyes when I recall it.

One of our fellow interns had been on call the 36 hours prior and was just finishing her shift. She was sleep deprived, mentally drained, and exhausted. All of which made her a prime target for Dr. A.

Dr A. began his sly scene with calling this unfortunate intern on the phone, imitating one of our attendings. "Intern, the reason for my call is to inform you that you did an excellent job with caring for Five of the admissions you admitted last night, however concerning the gentleman you admitted with septic shock, I have one very pressing question. Why did you not give the gamma? Did you even consider giving the gamma? The one thing that could save this patient's life, would be the gamma. I see that you did not give it? Please tell me this was a nursing order mistake. You did plan on giving the gamma, did you not Intern?

The intern looked like a deer in the headlights, soon to be replaced by a look of true terror. She was racking her fatigued brain for a shred of possibility to help her explain why indeed she had not given this life saving treatment. Thinking of gamma globulin? IVIG? Either of which would be completely inappropriate for septic shock. She uttered "The gamma? Uh, yes we considered giving the gamma. We have not given the gamma yet."

Dr. A returned, " Well why the hell not? Are you going to give the gamma?"

The intern replied, "Of course sir, I will give the gamma immediately."

After hanging up, Dr. A walked into the room this

distraught intern was standing in. Without cracking a smile, Dr. A. asked the intern, are you alright? You look upset. The intern replied, "I have to give the gamma. I know I have to give it. How do I write the order for the gamma?"

Dr. A. replied, "Just write..**THE GAMMA**." At that point the entire room broke apart with laughter. Some sympathetic soul informed the intern that the gamma was a fictitious medication and that she had been on the receiving end of another of Dr. A's pranks. The intern burst out in tears and left the room.

Although that intern was upset at Dr. A for a while, Dr. A taught us all a very important lesson that day. When you become a physician, you have people's lives depending on you. You have many pressures upon you, with many differing opinions from both physicians and patients. There are life saving treatments to give, but if you are administering a treatment that you do not fully understand, that you are not fully certain of, you are risking much more to your patient than doing nothing at all.

Always remember "Primum Non Nocere." (First Do No Harm)

There is Solice in Having Your Peeps

The medical field is isolating. It can be depressing. It is difficult to explain to those who have not endured the hardship. However, providers in the same field tend to lean on one another heavily. "Misery loves company" is the term.

The group doctors train with, are not only peers, but they soon become extended family. The group spends more time with each other than with their own respective nuclear families. Hours are long and strong bonds are formed. Doctors get each other's jokes. They have passive-aggressive cynicism, that at many times, only they find funny. Commonly, the jokes are dark, but humor allows a little light in.

HIPPA is another important factor to consider. Doctors are not able to discuss patient's conditions or cases outside of the hospital/clinic, nor outside of the patient's field of treatment. This additional constraint makes coping difficult for doctors. Experiencing loss on a daily basis is the norm, and it is difficult for most other people to relate.

This accentuates the importance of "having your peeps". Your peeps are other doctors that can weigh in on difficult medical decisions focused around patient care. Your peeps understand the anguish and turmoil associated with medical decision-making and what it means as a human being to accept as a doctor. Your peeps understand loss and triumph. Your peeps are irreplaceable. When one or more is lost, it is difficult to explain the level of disparity.

To my peeps, Doctors FG, HF, TT, IB, AO, AA, JP, PJ, TA, and RK, JS, JL, KK, SI, SK, I salute you. Thank you for your enduring dedication to making this world a better place, one patient at a time. In addition, I thank you for being a part of my extraordinary family.

No matter the field of medicine, there is solice in having your peeps.

The Most Beautiful
Thing I Ever Saw

Learning an additional language is fun and extremely helpful should you run into a patient from another country. It is true, a Spanish speaker is the most common patient you will cross paths with, however Spanish is not the only language which is useful to learn.

As a resident, I remember having a patient on my service who spoke only German. She and her husband had been traveling from Germany for vacation when she experienced an acute hemorrhagic stroke. Serendipitously, I had taken some German myself and was able to speak some with them, so they could understand what was going on, without the use of a poorly receptioned, telephone translator.

I met daily with this couple and updated them

as to the patients' status and plan. Unfortunately, secondary to the stroke, the patient became unable to speak, and it became questionable regarding her full mental status at all. Her husband remained at her side, day after day. And although he was with his wife, he was also very alone.

As these two were from out of the country, transport and discharge was a much longer process than usual. Thus, this poor man settled in for a world in which he could not communicate. He did not understand treatments being given as he was not in the medical field, nor were the treatments the patient was receiving similar to those in Germany. Even with all of these obstacles, this man never left his wife's side. Day after day, he would come and sit in her room at her bedside. Week after week he proved his undying loyalty.

It was not until I had a night on call with this unfortunate couple that my life was changed irrefutably. I had been called by one of the nurses on the neuro floor to come and evaluate "a sick patient". Reportedly the patient had become quite somnolent and was unarousable. As I rushed to the floor I found this patient to be my little German woman.

I quickly ordered a stat EKG, CXR, Troponin I, and a repeat head CT. The first thing to return was an EKG with severe tumbstoning. I remember thinking to myself, this woman has experienced an acute hemorrhagic head bleed, please don't have an MI…. However, that is exactly what she had.

I transferred my little German woman to the ICU, I intubated her, and placed a central line. I gave her absolutely nothing to combat her acute MI, as everything I would give her to protect her heart would either worsen her head bleed or drop her blood pressure. As a matter of fact, I had to give her medications which worsened and extended her MI to keep her blood pressure from bottoming out. I called her husband, who was staying at a very cheap motel 1 mile from the hospital to inform him of her change in condition. I remember him telling me he would be right down.

In 10 minutes, he was at his wife's bedside, as he had run on foot from his hotel, through a very dangerous neighborhood, at 1:00am! He was covered in sweat, tears were pouring down his face, mucous streamed from his nose, when he asked me, " Doctor Y, is my wife going to die?"

I grabbed a tissue box and began to explain the complex situation. When I was finished my little German man did something I had never seen before. He stumbled over to his wife, intubated, with blood on her chest from her central line placement. She was covered with wires and tubes and she was completely indiscernible from her previous appearance. He began to kiss her all over. He kissed her forehead, he kissed her cheek, he kissed her mouth around the endotracheal tube. In between his kisses he was telling her,"I love you, don't be afraid. I love you, don't be afraid. I love you don't be afraid. I am here with you and I will never leave you. You are not alone."

This continued until my little German woman passed, never waking, never struggling, never alone.

About the Author

After graduating medical school from San Francisco, California, then completing residency in Las Vegas, Nevada, Dr. Y. is roughly a 20-year medical veteran. Dr. Y. continues to actively practice, board certified in Internal Medicine and Hospitalist Medicine.

Printed in the United States
by Baker & Taylor Publisher Services